MW01231963

THE COMPLETE BREAD MACHINE COOKBOOK

An Easy-To-Follow Cookbook To Bake Amazing Recipes That Wow Your Family And Your Friends

By
Caren Cooper

Copyright © 2021

All rights reserved. No part of this publication may be reproduced or distributed in any form or by any means, electronic or mechanical, photocopying, scanning, recording or otherwise, without prior written permission from the publisher and the author.

Disclaimer of Warranty / Limit of Liability: The author and the publisher are not a licensed physician, medical professional or practitioner and offers no medical counseling, treatments or diagnoses. The author and the publisher make no warranties with respect to the accuracy and completeness of the contents of this work. All the nutritional facts contained in this book is provided for informational purposes only. The information is based on the specific ingredients, measurements and brands used to make the recipe. Therefore, the nutritional facts in this work in no way is intended to be a guarantee of the actual nutritional value of the recipe made by the reader. The author and the publisher will not be responsible for any damages resulting in reliance of the reader on the nutritional information.

The content presented herein, has not been evaluated by the U.S. Food and Drug Administration, and it is not intended to cure or diagnose any disease. This book isn't intended as a substitute for medical advice as physicians. Full medical clearance from a licensed physician should be obtained before beginning any diet. The advice and strategies contained herein may not be suitable for every situation. Neither the author nor the publisher claims no responsibility to any person or entity for any liability, damage or loss caused directly or indirectly as a result of the use, application or interpretation of the information presented in this work.

The publisher publishes its books in a variety of print and electronic formats. Some content that appears in print may not be available in electronic, and vice versa.

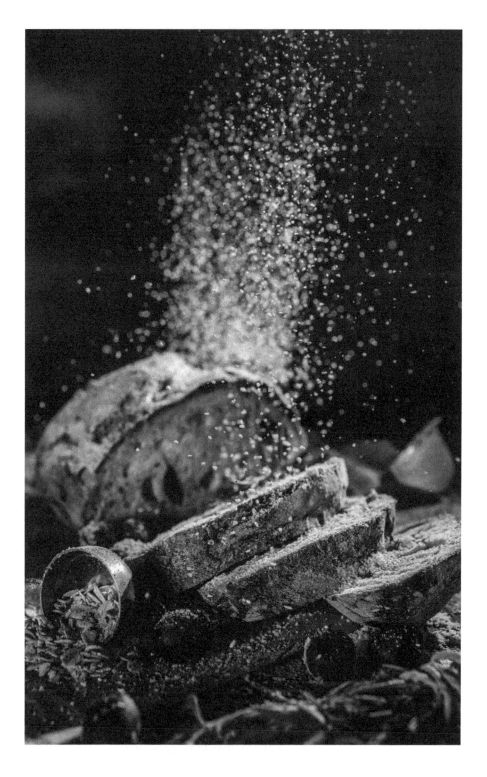

Table Of Contents

INTRODUCTION 8

CHAPTER 1: HOW TO BAKE USING A BREAD MACHINE.................10

CHAPTER 2: HOW TO USE A BREAD MACHINE 12

MEET YOUR NEW BREAD MACHINE.. 12
MAIN INGREDIENTS.. 13

CHAPTER 3: WHAT ARE THE MOST COMMON INGREDIENTS........16

CHAPTER 4: TIPS AND TRICKS IN ORDER TO HAVE A BETTER
FINAL PRODUCT AND TO SAVE MONEY AND TIME 20

CHAPTER 5: PERFECT FOR BREAKFAST 26

1.   FLUFFY PALEO BREAD 26

CHAPTER 6: WHOLE-WHEAT BREAD 28

2.   BUTTERMILK WHEAT BREAD.. 28

CHAPTER 7: CLASSIC BREAD 30

3.   WHITE BREAD.. 30

CHAPTER 8: SPICE AND HERB BREAD 32

4. SAFFRON TOMATO BREAD 32

CHAPTER 9: SOURDOUGH BREAD 34

5. HONEY SOURDOUGH BREAD.. 34

CHAPTER 10: SWEET BREAD 36

6. CHOCOLATE CHIP PEANUT BUTTER BANANA BREAD................... 36
7. CHOCOLATE SOUR CREAM BREAD 38

CHAPTER 11: CHEESE BREAD 40

8. BLUE CHEESE ONION BREAD... 40
9. CHEESE LOAF.. 42

CHAPTER 12: DOUGH RECIPES 44

10. CHOCOLATE ZUCCHINI BREAD... 44

CHAPTER 13: BUNS & BREAD **46**

11.   MUSTARD BEER BREAD 46

CHAPTER 14: BREAD MACHINE RECIPES **48**

12.   DUTCH OVEN BREAD 48
13.   ARTICHOKE BREAD 50

CHAPTER 15: NUT AND SEED BREAD **52**

14.   CHERRY AND ALMOND BREAD 52
15.   NUTTY WHEAT BREAD 54

CHAPTER 16: VEGETABLE BREAD **56**

16.   HEALTHY CELERY LOAF 56
17.   BROCCOLI AND CAULIFLOWER BREAD 58

CHAPTER 17: BASIC BREAD **60**

18.   ANADAMA BREAD 60

CHAPTER 18: PLEASURE BREAD **62**

19.   HONEY BEER BREAD 62

CHAPTER 19: CAKES AND QUICK BREAD **64**

20.   CINNAMON PECAN COFFEE CAKE 64

CHAPTER 20: MEAT BREAD **66**

21.   COLLARDS & BACON GRILLED PIZZA 66

CHAPTER 21: MULTI-GRAIN BREAD **68**

22.   BAGUETTE STYLE FRENCH BREAD 68

CHAPTER 22: HOLIDAY BREAD **72**

23.   RAISIN CINNAMON SWIRL BREAD 72

CHAPTER 23: KETO BREAD RECIPES **76**

24.   GREAT FLAVOR CHEESE BREAD WITH THE ADDED KICK OF PIMENTO OLIVES 76
25.   RICOTTA CHIVE BREAD 78
26.   RED HOT CINNAMON BREAD 79

CHAPTER 24: INTERNATIONAL BREAD **82**

27.   SWEDISH CARDAMOM BREAD 82

CHAPTER 25: FRUIT AND VEGETABLE BREAD 84

28.   BLUEBERRY BREAD 84
29.   PINEAPPLE COCONUT BREAD 86

CHAPTER 26: WHITE BREAD 88

30.   SOFT WHITE BREAD 88

CHAPTER 27: SPECIAL BREAD RECIPES 90

31.   GLUTEN-FREE PEASANT BREAD 90
32.   GLUTEN-FREE HAWAIIAN LOAF 92

CHAPTER 28: ROLLS AND PIZZA 94

33.   CHEESE STUFFED GARLIC ROLLS 94

CHAPTER 29: ITALIAN STYLED 96

34.   VEGGIE LOAF 96
35.   CAJUN VEGGIE LOAF 98
36.   PARMESAN ITALIAN BREAD 100

CHAPTER 30: FAMOUS BREAD RECIPES 102

37.   BEST KETO BREAD 102
38.   BREAD DE SOUL 104
39.   CHIA SEED BREAD 106
40.   SPECIAL KETO BREAD 108

CONCLUSION 110

CONVERSION TABLES 112

MEASURING EQUIVALENT CHART 112
GLUTEN-FREE – CONVERSION TABLES 114
FLOUR: QUANTITY AND WEIGHT 115
SUGAR: QUANTITY AND WEIGHT 115
CREAM: QUANTITY AND WEIGHT 116
BUTTER: QUANTITY AND WEIGHT 116
OVEN TEMPERATURE EQUIVALENT CHART 117

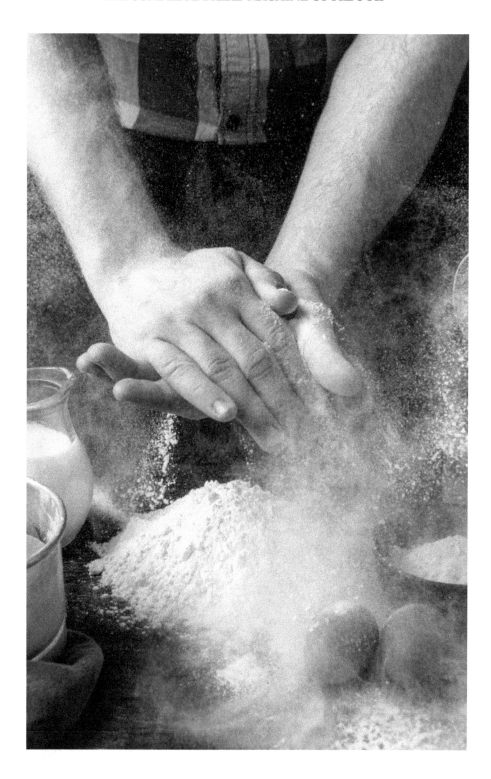

Introduction

To bake bread, ingredients are measured in a specified order into the bread pan (usually first liquids, with solid ingredients layered on top), and then the pan is put in the bread maker. The order of ingredients is important because contact with water triggers the instant yeast used in bread makers, so the yeast and water have to be kept separate until the program starts.

It takes the machine several hours to make a bread loaf. The products are rested first and brought to an optimal temperature. Stir with a paddle, and the ingredients are then shaped into flour.

Use optimal temperature regulation, and the dough is then confirmed and then cooked.

When the bread has been baked, the bread maker removes the pan. Then leaving a slight indentation from the rod to which the paddle is connected. The finished loaf's shape is often regarded as unique.

Many initial bread machines manufacture a vertically slanted towards, square, or cylindrical loaf that is significantly dissimilar from commercial bread; however, more recent units typically have a more conventional horizontal pan. Some bread machines use two paddles to form two lb. loaf in regular rectangle shape.

Bread makers are also fitted with a timer for testing when bread-making starts. For example, this allows them to be loaded at night but only begin baking in the morning to produce a freshly baked bread for breakfast.

They may also be set only for making dough, for example, for making pizza.

Apart from bread, some can also be set to make other things like jam, pasta dough, and Japanese rice cake. Some of the new developments in the facility of the machine includes automatically adding nut.

It also contains fruit from a tray during the kneading process. Bread makers typically take between three and four hours to bake a loaf. However, recent "quick bake" modes have become standard additions, many of which can produce a loaf in less than an hour.

CHAPTER 1:

How to Bake Using a Bread Machine

The flour is run to cover the liquid layer entirely, and then different dry ingredients are poured. Salt, sugar, hard butter (butter) is placed in the grooves made in the stacked layers to not come into contact with each other.

Then, in the middle of the dry components layer, depression is caused, and yeast is poured into it (the depression should not reach the liquid coating).

A container with food is placed in the oven (usually there are special fasteners), the lid is closed, and the oven is plugged into a power outlet. Choose a program, the finished product's size, and the crust (if provided in the model). Press the "Start" or "Start" button. After that, the kneading process begins. If the oven has a timer, then you can set the time for preparing the bread for a specific time.

During kneading, the dough is checked by periodically opening the lid. To make good bread, the dough should be slightly sticky to the touch. If the dough is too soft and moist, add a little flour; if it turns out to be very dense, add liquid.

It is essential to assess the state of the dough during the lifting process. The dough may rise too high on hot days, and then it falls out of the mold and falls on the heating coils.

To not change the baking program, the dough can be punctured in several places to fall off. Or, cancel the originally specified program and set the mode, which in many models is called "Baking only."

All additives fall asleep after the stove signal about the end of the kneading, also, by a timer indicating that the kneading process is completed. If the stove has an automatic addition mode, then all components are poured into a special compartment at the beginning of cooking, as we have already mentioned earlier.

At the end of the cycle, the bread maker beeps. It either turns off itself in automatic mode, or you should press the "Stop" button. After that, the lid is opened, gloves are put on. The bread is then taken out (it is not recommended to lean close to the open stove and also rely on it).

CHAPTER 2:

How to Use a Bread Machine

Meet Your New Bread Machine

Even if you're not good at using modern appliances, put your worries behind you, because bread machines have simple, easy-to-use controls.

They are fun and easy to use! Besides making fresh bread, they can also make and knead any type of dough, bake dough out of the box, and even make dough jam. When you get to know this handy device, it will truly become an essential and exceptional aid in your kitchen.

It's so simple

Insert the baking sheet into the machine.

Attach the dough blades.

Add ingredients as shown in your machine manual.

Close the lid.

Turn on the machine.

Select the required function.

What Else Can It Do?

Different bread machines may differ in their design, capacity, number of accessories, and programs available. When choosing your bread machine, think of your own preferences and needs: What will you do with the machine? Do you need any particular programs and additional modes, or is the basic functionality enough?

Bread machines can knead the dough, let it rest, bake a crunchy baguette, make sweet cupcakes or unleavened bread, and much more.

Main Ingredients

There are other ingredients that add flavor, texture, and nutrition to your bread, such as sugar, fats, and eggs. The basic ingredients include:

Flour is the foundation of bread.

The protein and gluten in flour forms a network that traps the carbon dioxide and alcohol produced by the yeast. Flour also provides simple sugar to feed the yeast and it provides flavor, depending on the type of flour used in the recipe.

Yeast is a living organism that increases when the right amount of moisture, food, and heat are applied. Rapidly multiplying yeast gives off carbon dioxide and ethyl alcohol.

When yeast is allowed to go through its life cycle completely, the finished bread is more flavorful.

The best yeast for bread machines is bread machine yeast or active dry yeast, depending on your bread machine model.

Salt strengthens gluten and slows the rise of the bread by retarding the action of the yeast. A slower rise allows the flavors of the bread to develop better, and it will be less likely the bread will rise too much.

Liquid activates the yeast and dissolves the other ingredients. The most commonly used liquid is water, but ingredients such as milk can also be substituted. Bread made with water will have a crisper crust, but milk produces rich, tender bread that offers more nutrition and browns easier.

Oils and fats add flavor, create a tender texture, and help brown the crust. Bread made with fat stays fresh longer because moisture loss in the bread is slowed. This component can also inhibit gluten formation, so the bread does not rise as high.

Sugar is the source of food for the yeast. It also adds sweetness, tenderness, and color to the crust. Too much sugar can inhibit gluten growth or cause the dough to rise too much and collapse. Other sweeteners can replace sugar, such as honey, molasses, maple syrup, brown sugar, and corn syrup.

Eggs add protein, flavor, color, and a tender crust. Eggs contain an emulsifier, lecithin, which helps create a consistent texture, and a leavening agent, which helps the bread rise well.

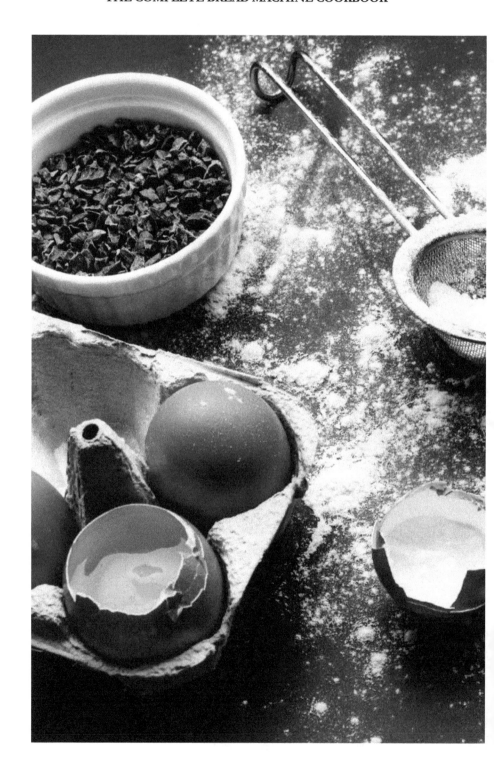

CHAPTER 3:

What are the Most Common Ingredients

Knowing the role of these ingredients helps you to understand the baking process. Moreover, the order in which you add ingredients is crucial when making bread in your bread machine.

Water/Milk

All of the other basic bread ingredients, including flour, salt, and yeast, need a liquid medium to do their respective tasks. Water is the most common liquid ingredient; milk, buttermilk, cream, and juice are some common substitutes.

The liquid is usually the first ingredient to be added to the bread pan. This is very important as it maintains the ideal texture of your bread. The liquid should not be cold; ensure that it is lukewarm (between 80 and 90°F) whenever possible.

Sugar/honey (if using)

Sweet ingredients such as honey, corn syrup, maple syrup, and sugar are usually added after the butter as they mix easily with water and butter. However, the sweetener can be added before the butter as well. Sugar, honey, etc. serve as a feeding medium for yeast, so fermentation is stronger with the addition of sweet ingredients.

Eggs (if using)

Eggs need to be at room temperature before they are added to the bread pan. If the eggs are taken from the refrigerator, keep them outside at room temperature until they are no longer cold. They keep the crust tender and add protein and flavor to the bread.

Chilled Ingredients

If you are using any other ingredient that is kept chilled, such as cheese, milk, buttermilk or cream, keep it outside at room temperature until it is no longer cold, or microwave it for a few seconds to warm it up.

Salt

Use table salt or non-iodized salt for better results. Salt that is high in iodine can hamper the activity of the yeast and create problems with fermentation.

Furthermore, salt itself is a yeast inhibitor and should not be touching yeast directly; that is why salt and yeast are never added together or one after another.

Flour

Flour is the primary ingredient for any bread recipe. It contains gluten (except for the gluten-free flours) and protein, and when the yeast produces alcohol and carbon dioxide, the gluten and protein trap the alcohol and carbon dioxide to initiate the bread-making process.

There are many different types of flours used for preparing different types of bread. Bread machine flour or white bread flour is the most common type as it is suitable for most bread recipes.

Seeds (if using)

If a recipe calls for adding seeds such as sunflower seeds or caraway seeds, these should be added after the flour. However, when two different flours are being used, it is best to add the seeds in between the flours for a better mix.

Yeast

Yeast is the ingredient responsible for initiating the vital bread-making process of fermentation. Yeast needs the right amount of heat, moisture and liquid to grow and multiply. When yeast multiplies, it releases alcohol and carbon dioxide.

You can use active dry yeast or bread machine yeast (both will be available in local grocery stores). Cool, dry places are ideal to store yeast packs.

Yeast is added to the bread pan last, after the flour and other dry ingredients. (For certain types of bread, like fruit and nut bread, yeast is technically not the last ingredient, as the fruits or nuts are added later by the machine.

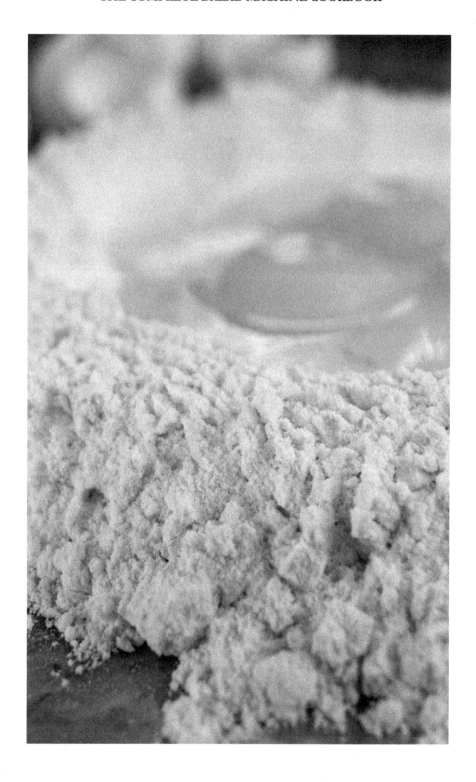

CHAPTER 4:

Tips and tricks in Order to have a Better Final Product and to Save Money and Time

When you are using a bread machine for the first time, it's common to have some concerns. However, they are quite easy to fix.

The following are some useful tips and quick-and-easy fixes for the most common problems encountered while baking bread in a bread machine.

Dough Check

You can check the progress of the dough while the bread machine is mixing the ingredients. Take a quick check after 5 minutes of kneading. An ideal dough with the right amount of dry and wet ingredients makes one smooth ball and feels slightly tacky.

You can open the lid to evaluate the dough. Do not worry about interfering with the kneading process by opening the lid; the bread structure won't be affected even if you poke it to get a feel for the dough.

If the dough feels too wet/moist or does not form into a ball shape, you can add 1 tablespoon of flour at a time and check again after a few minutes. If you feel that the dough is too dry, or it has formed two or three small balls, you can add 1 teaspoon of water at a time and check again after a few minutes.

Fruit/Nut Bread

When making fruit or nut bread, it is very important to add fruits or nuts at the right time. Not all bread machines come with a nut/fruit dispenser or hopper. If yours doesn't have one, don't worry; the machine will signal you with a beep series when it's time to add the fruits or nuts.

Citrus Ingredients

Citrus ingredients such as lemon zest, orange zest, orange juice, lemon juice, and pineapple juice can create issues with yeast fermentation if added in excess. Do not add more than the quantity specified in a recipe. The same goes for alcohol and cinnamon.

Salt Adjustment

When making small loaves (around 1 pound), sometimes the loaf rises more or less than expected. In many such instances, the issue is with the quantity of salt added. To avoid problems, try using less salt or cutting back on the quantity specified in the recipe. Using sea salt or coarse salt can also help prevent problems with small loaves.

Bread Collapse

The amount of yeast is very important for proper rising. The most common reason for bread collapse during the baking process is adding too much or too little yeast. Do not add more yeast than specified in the recipe. Also, check the expiration date on the yeast pack; freshly packed yeast provides the best results. Other reasons for bread collapse are using cold water and adding excess salt.

Failure to Rise

Many factors can contribute to the failure of dough to rise completely. Insufficient gluten content, miscalculated ingredients, excess salt, excess sugar, and using cold ingredients are the most common reasons. Always warm any chilled ingredients or place them at room temperature for a while before adding them to the bread pan. However, if you are warming any ingredients in your oven, make sure not to overheat them. They need to be lukewarm, at between 80 and 90°F, and not too hot. Also make sure that the yeast does not come in direct contact with the salt, as this creates problems with rising (that is why yeast is added last).

Texture Troubles

- If your bread has a coarse texture, try adding more salt and reducing the amount of liquid.

- If your bread looks small and feels dense, try using flour with higher protein content. Bread flour has a sufficient amount of protein, but slightly denser loaves are common when you use heavier flours such as rye flour and whole wheat flour. Use additional ingredients such as fruits, nuts, and vegetables in their specified quantities. Adding too much of such ingredients will make your loaf too heavy, small, and dense.

- Moist or gummy loaves are less common, but it can happen if you have added too much liquid or used too much sugar. Too much liquid can also result in a doughy center.

- If your bread has an unbrowned top, try adding more sugar. This can also happen if your bread machine has a glass top.

- If your loaf has a mushroom top, it is probably due to too much yeast or water. Try reducing the amount of water and/or yeast.

- Sometimes a baked loaf has some flour on one side. When you bake the next time, try to remove any visible flour during the kneading cycle with a rubber spatula.

- If your loaf has an overly dark crust, try using the Medium crust setting next time. This also happens if you've added too much sugar and when you fail to take out the bread pan after the end of the baking process. It is always advisable to remove the bread pan right after the process is complete.

- If your loaf has a sunken top, it is probably because of using too much liquid or overly hot ingredients. This is also common during humid or warm weather.

Excess Rise

Many times, a loaf rises more than expected; the most common reasons are too much yeast, too little salt, and using cold water. But also make sure that the capacity of your bread pan is sufficient for the size of loaf you have selected; trying to make a large loaf in a small bread pan will obviously lead to such trouble.

Paddles

After the bread machine completes its baking process the paddles may remain inside the bread loaf. Allow the freshly made bread to cool down and then place it on a cutting board and gently take out the paddles.

Spraying the paddles with a cooking spray before you add the ingredients to the bread pan will make it easier to clean them after the bread is baked.

Cleaning

After you take the baked loaf from the bread pan, do not immerse the pan in water. Rather, fill it with warm soapy water.

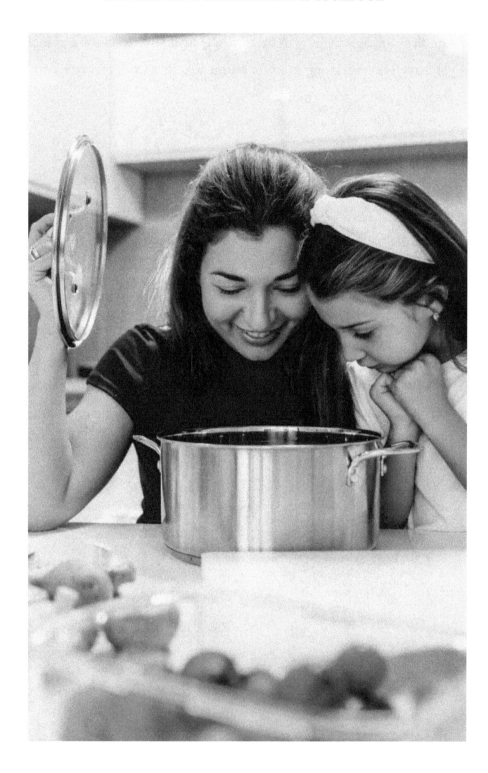

CHAPTER 5:

Perfect for Breakfast

1.   Fluffy Paleo Bread

Preparation Time: 10 minutes

Cooking Time: 40 minutes

Servings: 15

Ingredients:

- One ¼ cup almond flour
- Five eggs
- 1 tsp. lemon juice
- 1/3 cup avocado oil
- One dash black pepper
- ½ tsp. sea salt
- 3 to 4 tbsp. tapioca flour
- 1 to 2 tsp. Poppyseed
- ¼ cup ground flaxseed
- ½ tsp. baking soda
- Top with:

- Poppy seeds

- Pumpkin seeds

Directions:

1. Preheat the oven to 350F.

2. Line a baking pan with parchment paper and set aside.

3. In a bowl, add eggs, avocado oil, and lemon juice and whisk until combined.

4. In another bowl, add tapioca flour, almond flour, baking soda, flaxseed, black pepper, and poppy seed. Mix.

5. Add the lemon juice mixture into the flour mixture and mix well.

6. Add the batter into the prepared loaf pan and top with extra pumpkin seeds and poppy seeds.

7. Cover loaf pan and transfer into the prepared oven, and bake for 20 minutes. Remove cover and bake until an inserted knife comes out clean after about 15 to 20 minutes.

8. Remove from oven and cool. Slice and serve.

Nutrition:

Calories: 149 Cal

Fat: 12.9 g

Carbohydrates: 4.4 g

CHAPTER 6:

Whole-Wheat Bread

2.   Buttermilk Wheat Bread

Preparation Time: 8 Minutes

Cooking Time: 4 Hours and 30 Minutes

Servings: 16 slices

Ingredients:

- Buttermilk, at room temperature
- White sugar
- Olive oil
- Salt
- Baking soda
- Unbleached white flour
- Whole wheat flour
- Active dry yeast

Directions:

1. In the bread machine pan, measure all ingredients in the order the manufacturer recommends.

2. Set the machine to the Basic White Bread setting and press START.

3. After a few minutes, add more buttermilk if the ingredients don't form a ball. If it's too loose, apply a handful of flour.

4. One baked, let the bread cool on a wire rack before slicing.

5. Enjoy!

Nutrition:

Calories: 141

Carbs: 26g

Fat: 2.5g

Protein: 5g

<h1 style="text-align:center">CHAPTER 7:</h1>

Classic Bread

3.   White Bread

Preparation Time: 5 Minutes

Cooking Time: 3 Hours and 5 Minutes

Servings: 8

Ingredients:

- 1 cup of lukewarm water (110 degrees F/45 degrees C)
- Three tablespoons of white sugar
- 1 1/2 teaspoons of salt
- Three tablespoons of vegetable oil
- 3 cups of bread flour
- 2 1/4 teaspoons of active dry yeast

Directions:

1. Put water, sugar, salt, oil, bread flour, and yeast into the bread machine.

2. Bake on setting White Bread. Before slicing, let it cool on wire racks.

Nutrition:

Carbohydrates 3 g

Fats 5.6 g

Protein 9.6 g

Calories 319

CHAPTER 8:

Spice and Herb Bread

4. Saffron Tomato Bread

Preparation Time: 3 hours 30 minutes

Cooking Time: 15 minutes

Servings: 10

Ingredients:

- 1 teaspoon bread machine yeast
- 2½ cups wheat bread machine flour
- 1 Tablespoon panifarin
- 1½ teaspoon kosher salt
- 1½ Tablespoon white sugar
- Tablespoon extra-virgin olive oil
- Tablespoon tomatoes, dried and chopped
- 1 Tablespoon tomato paste
- ½ cup firm cheese (cubes)
- ½ cup feta cheese
- 1 pinch saffron
- 1½ cups serum

Directions:

1 Five minutes before cooking, pour in dried tomatoes and 1 tablespoon of olive oil. Add the tomato paste and mix.

2 Place all the dry and liquid ingredients, except additives, in the pan and follow the instructions for your bread machine.

3 Pay particular attention to measuring the ingredients. Use a measuring cup, measuring spoon, and kitchen scales to do so.

4 Set the baking program to BASIC and the crust type to MEDIUM.

5 Add the additives after the beep or place them in the dispenser of the bread machine.

6 Shake the loaf out of the pan. If necessary, use a spatula.

7 Wrap the bread with a kitchen towel and set it aside for an hour. Otherwise, you can cool it on a wire rack.

Nutrition:

Calories: 260 calories;

Total Carbohydrate: 35.5 g

Cholesterol: 20 g

Total Fat: 9.2g

Protein: 8.9 g

Sodium: 611 mg

Sugar: 5.2 g

CHAPTER 9:

Sourdough Bread

5. Honey Sourdough Bread

Preparation Time: 15 minutes; 1 week (Starter)

Cooking Time: 3 hours

Servings: 1 loaf

Ingredients:

- 2/3 cup sourdough starter
- 1/2 cup water
- 1 tablespoon vegetable oil
- tablespoons honey
- 1/2 teaspoon salt
- 1/2 cup high protein wheat flour
- cups bread flour
- 1 teaspoon active dry yeast

Directions:

1 Measure 1 cup of starter and remaining bread ingredients, add to bread machine pan.

2 Choose basic/white bread cycle with medium or light crust color.

Nutrition:

Calories: 175 calories;

Total Carbohydrate: 33 g

Total Fat: 0.3 g

Protein: 5.6 g

Sodium: 121 mg

Fiber: 1.9 g

CHAPTER 10:

Sweet Bread

6. Chocolate Chip Peanut Butter Banana Bread

Preparation Time: 25 Minutes

Cooking Time: 10 Minutes

Servings: 12 to 16 slices

Ingredients:

- Two bananas, mashed
- Two eggs, at room temperature
- 1/2 cup melted butter, cooled
- Two tablespoons milk, at room temperature
- One teaspoon pure vanilla extract
- cups all-purpose flour
- 1/2 cup sugar
- 11/4 teaspoons baking powder
- 1/2 teaspoon baking soda
- 1/2 teaspoon salt
- 1/2 cup peanut butter chips
- 1/2 cup semisweet chocolate chips

Directions:

1   Stir together the bananas, eggs, butter, milk, and vanilla in the bread machine bucket and set it aside.

2   In a medium bowl, toss together the flour, sugar, baking powder, baking soda, salt, peanut butter chips, and chocolate chips.

3   Add the dry ingredients to the bucket.

4   Program the machine for Quick/Rapid bread, and press Start.

5   When the cake is made, stick a knife into it, and if it arises out clean, the loaf is done.

6   If the loaf needs a few more minutes, look at the management panel for a Bake Only button, and extend the time by 10 minutes.

7   When the loaf is done, remove the bucket from the machine.

8   Let the loaf cool for 5 minutes.

9   Gently rock the can to remove the bread and turn it out onto a rack to cool.

Nutrition:

Calories: 297

Total Fat: 14g

Saturated Fat: 7g

Carbohydrates: 40g

Fiber: 1g

Sodium: 255mg

Protein: 4g

7. Chocolate Sour Cream Bread

Preparation Time: 25 Minutes

Cooking Time: 10 Minutes

Servings: 12 slices

Ingredients:

- 1 cup sour cream
- Two eggs, at room temperature
- 1 cup of sugar
- 1/2 cup (1 stick) butter, at room temperature
- 1/4 cup plain Greek yogurt
- 13/4 cups all-purpose flour
- 1/2 cup unsweetened cocoa powder
- 1/2 teaspoon baking powder
- 1/2 teaspoon salt
- 1 cup milk chocolate chips

Directions:

1 In a small bowl, stick together the sour cream, eggs, sugar, butter, and yogurt until just combined.
2 Transfer the wet ingredients to the bread machine bucket, and then add the flour, cocoa powder, baking powder, salt, and chocolate chips.
3 Program the machine for Quick/Rapid bread, and press Start.

4   When the loaf is done, stick a knife into it, and if it comes out clean, the loaf is done.

5   If the loaf needs a few more minutes, check the control panel for a Bake Only button and extend the time by 10 minutes.

6   When the loaf is done, remove the bucket from the machine.

7   Let the loaf cool for 5 minutes.

8   Gently rock the can to remove the loaf and place it out onto a rack to cool.

Nutrition:

Calories: 347

Total Fat: 16g

Saturated Fat: 9g

Carbohydrates: 48g

Fiber: 2g

Sodium: 249mg

Protein: 6g

CHAPTER 11:

Cheese Bread

8. Blue Cheese Onion Bread

Preparation Time: 10 Minutes

Cooking Time: 25 Minutes

Servings: 8

Ingredients:

- 1¼ cup water, at 80°F to 90°F

- One egg, at room temperature

- One tablespoon melted butter cooled

- ¼ cup powdered skim milk

- One tablespoon sugar

- ¾ teaspoon salt

- ½ cup (2 ounces) crumbled blue cheese

- One tablespoon dried onion flake

- 3 cups white bread flour

- ¼ cup instant mashed potato flakes

- One teaspoon bread machine or active dry yeast

Directions:

1. Preparing the Ingredients. Place the ingredients in your Zojirushi bread machine.

2. Program the machine for Regular Basic, select light or medium crust, and press Start.

3. Remove the bucket from the machine.

4. Let the loaf cool for 5 minutes.

5. Gently shake the container to remove the loaf and turn it out onto a rack to cool.

Nutrition:

Calories 174

Carbs 31.1g

Fat 3.1g

Protein 5.1g

9. Cheese Loaf

Preparation Time: 10 Minutes

Cooking Time: 25 Minutes

Servings: 8

Ingredients:

- 1/4 cups flour
- tsp. instant yeast
- 1 3/4 cups water
- tbsp. sugar
- 1 1/2 cup shredded cheddar cheese
- tbsp. parmesan cheese
- 1 tsp. mustard
- 1 tsp. paprika
- tbsp. minced white onion
- 1/3 cup butter

Directions:

1   Begin through placing all ingredients in the bread pan in the liquid-dry-yeast layering.
2   Put the pan in the Zojirushi bread machine.
3   Select the Bake cycle. Choose Regular Basic Setting and light crust.
4   Press start and wait until the loaf is cooked.

5   The machine will start the keep warm mode after the bread is complete.

6   For about 10 minutes, let the bread stay for 10 minutes in that mode before unplugging.

7   You may now want to remove the pan and let it cool down for about 10 minutes.

Nutrition:

Calories 174

Carbs 31.1g

Fat 3.1g

Protein 5.1g

CHAPTER 12:

Dough Recipes

10. Chocolate Zucchini Bread

Preparation Time: 10 minutes

Cooking Time: 20 minutes

Servings: 10

Ingredients:

- cups grated zucchini, excess moisture removed
- eggs
- Tbsp. olive oil
- 1/3 cup low-carb sweetener
- 1 tsp. vanilla extract
- 1/3 cup coconut flour
- ¼ cup unsweetened cocoa powder
- ½ tsp. baking soda
- ½ tsp. salt
- 1/3 cup sugar-free chocolate chips

Directions:

1   Preheat the oven to 350F.

2   Grease the baking pan and line the entire pan with parchment paper.

3   In a food processor, blend the eggs, zucchini, oil, sweetener, and vanilla.

4   Add the flour, cocoa, baking soda, and salt to the zucchini mixture and stir until mixed. For a few seconds, let the batter sit.

5   Mix in the chocolate chips, then dispense the batter into the prepared pan.

6   Bake for 45 to 50 minutes.

7   Cool, slice, and serve.

Nutrition:

Calories: 149

Fat: 8g

Carb: 7g

Protein: 3g

CHAPTER 13:

Buns & Bread

11. Mustard Beer Bread

Preparation Time: 3 hours

Cooking Time: 0

Servings: 8

Ingredients:

- 1 ¼ cups dark beer
- 1/3 cups flour
- ¾ cup whole meal flour
- 1 tablespoon olive oil
- teaspoons mustard seeds
- 1 ½ teaspoons dry yeast
- 1 teaspoon salt
- teaspoons brown sugar

Directions:

1   Open a beer bottle and let it stand for 30 minutes to get out the gas.

2   In a bread maker's bucket, add the beer, mustard seeds, butter, sifted flour, and whole meal flour.

3   From different angles in the bucket, put salt and sugar. In the center of the flour, make a groove and fill with the mustard seeds.

4   Start the baking program.

Nutrition:

Carbohydrates 4.2 g

Fats 1 g

Protein 4.1 g

Calories 118

CHAPTER 14:

Bread machine recipes

12. Dutch Oven Bread

Preparation Time: 20 minutes

Cooking Time: 30 minutes

Servings: 6

Ingredients:

- 1 teaspoon baking powder
- 1 teaspoon baking soda
- cups almond flour
- 1 and ½ cups warm water
- A pinch of salt
- 1 teaspoon stevia

Directions:

1 Using a bowl, mix the water with the flour and stir well.

2 Add the rest of the ingredients, stir until you obtain a dough and leave aside for 20 minutes.

3   Transfer the dough to a dutch oven and bake the bread at 400 degrees f for 30 minutes.

4   Cool the bread down, slice and serve.

Nutrition:

Calories 143

Fat 9

Fiber 3

Carbs 4

Protein 6

13. Artichoke Bread

Preparation Time: 10 minutes

Cooking Time: 30 minutes

Servings: 10

Ingredients:

- oz. canned artichoke hearts
- 1 garlic clove, minced
- 1 cup parmesan, grated
- 1 cup almond flour
- ½ teaspoon baking powder
- 1 and ½ cups warm water

Directions:

1 Using a bowl, mix the flour with baking powder, and the water and stir well.
2 Add the rest of the ingredients, stir the dough well and transfer it to a lined round pan.
3 Bake at temperature 360 degrees f for 30 minutes, cool the bread down, slice and serve.

Nutrition:

Calories 211, Fat 12, Fiber 3, Carbs 5, Protein 6

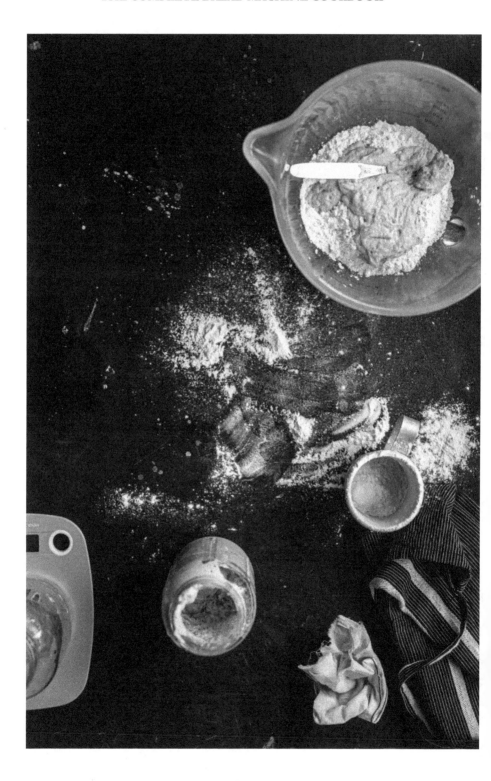

CHAPTER 15:

Nut and Seed Bread

14. Cherry and Almond Bread

Preparation Time: 10 Minutes

Cooking Time: 4 Hours

Servings: 8

Ingredients:

- Milk, lukewarm
- Butter, unsalted, softened
- Egg, at room temperature
- Bread flour
- Dried cherries
- Slivered almonds, toasted
- Salt
- Dry yeast, active
- Sugar

Directions:

1 Gather all the ingredients needed for the bread.

2 Power on bread machine that has about 2 pounds of the bread pan.

3   Add all the ingredients in the order mentioned in the ingredients list into the bread machine pan.

4   Press the "Dough" button, key the left button, and let mixture knead for 5 to 10 minutes.

5   Then select the "basic/white" down arrow to set baking time to 4 hours, select light or medium color for the crust, and press the start button.

6   Then prudently lift out the bread and put it on a wire rack for 1 hour or more until cooled.

7   Cut bread into sixteen slices and then serve.

Nutrition:

Calories: 125

Fat (g): 3

Protein (g): 4

Carbs: 20.4

15. Nutty Wheat Bread

Preparation Time: 10 Minutes

Cooking Time: 4 Hours

Servings: 12

Ingredients:

- Water, lukewarm
- Olive oil
- Honey
- Molasses
- Whole wheat flour
- Bread flour
- Dry yeast, active
- Salt
- Chopped pecans
- Chopped walnuts

Directions:

1   Gather all the ingredients needed for the bread.

2   Power on bread machine that has about 2 pounds of the bread pan.

3   Add all the ingredients in the order listed in the ingredients list into the bread machine pan except for pecans and nuts.

4 Press the "Dough" switch, press the start button, let mixture knead for 5 minutes, add pecans and nuts, and then continue kneading for another 5 minutes until all the ingredients have thoroughly combined and incorporated.

5 Then select the "basic/white" cycle, press the up/down arrow to make the baking time to 4 hours.

6 Select light or medium color for the crust, and press the start button.

7 Then put the bread on a wire rack for 1 hour or more until cooled.

8 Cut bread into twelve slices and then serve.

Nutrition:

Calories: 187

Fat (g): 7

Protein (g): 5

Carbs: 28

CHAPTER 16:

Vegetable Bread

16. Healthy Celery Loaf

Preparation Time: 2 hours 40 minutes

Cooking Time: 50 minutes

Servings: 1 loaf

Ingredients:

- 1 can (10 ounces) cream of celery soup
- tablespoons low-fat milk, heated
- 1 tablespoon vegetable oil
- 1¼ teaspoons celery salt
- ¾ cup celery, fresh/sliced thin
- 1 tablespoon celery leaves, fresh, chopped
- 1 whole egg
- ¼ teaspoon sugar
- cups bread flour
- ¼ teaspoon ginger
- ½ cup quick-cooking oats

- tablespoons gluten

- teaspoons celery seeds

- 1 pack of active dry yeast

Directions:

1   Add all of the ingredients to your bread machine, carefully following the instructions of the manufacturer

2   Set the program of your bread machine to Basic/White Bread and set crust type to Medium

3   Press START

4   Wait until the cycle completes

5   Once the loaf is ready, take the bucket out and let the loaf cool for 5 minutes

6   Gently shake the bucket to remove the loaf

7   Transfer to a cooling rack, slice and serve

8   Enjoy!

Nutrition:

Calories: 73 Cal

Fat: 4 g

Carbohydrates: 8 g

Protein: 3 g

Fiber: 1 g

17. Broccoli and Cauliflower Bread

Preparation Time: 2 hours 20 minutes

Cooking Time: 50 minutes

Servings: 1 loaf

Ingredients:

- ¼ cup water
- tablespoons olive oil
- 1 egg white
- 1 teaspoon lemon juice
- 2/3 cup grated cheddar cheese
- tablespoons green onion
- ½ cup broccoli, chopped
- ½ cup cauliflower, chopped
- ½ teaspoon lemon pepper seasoning
- cups bread flour
- 1 teaspoon bread machine yeast

Directions:

1   Add all of the ingredients to your bread machine, carefully following the instructions of the manufacturer

2   Set the program of your bread machine to Basic/White Bread and set crust type to Medium

3 Press START

4 Wait until the cycle completes

5 Once the loaf is ready, take the bucket out and let the loaf cool for 5 minutes

6 Gently shake the bucket to remove the loaf

7 Transfer to a cooling rack, slice and serve

8 Enjoy!

Nutrition:

Calories: 156 Cal

Fat: 8 g

Carbohydrates: 17 g

Protein: 5 g

Fiber: 2 g

CHAPTER 17:

Basic Bread

18.   Anadama Bread

Preparation Time: 3 hours

Cooking Time: 45 minutes

Servings: 2 loaves

Ingredients:

- 1/2 cup sunflower seeds

- Two teaspoons bread machine yeast

- 4 1/2 cups bread flour

- 3/4 cup yellow cornmeal

- Two tablespoons unsalted butter, cubed

- 1 1/2 teaspoon salt

- 1/4 cup dry skim milk powder

- 1/4 cup molasses

- 1 1/2 cups water, with a temperature of 80 to 90 degrees F (26 to 32 degrees C)

Directions:

1. Put all the pan's ingredients, except the sunflower seeds, in this order: water, molasses, milk, salt, butter, cornmeal, flour, and yeast.

2. Put the pan in the machine and cover the lid.

3. Put the sunflower seeds in the fruit and nut dispenser.

4. Turn the machine on and choose the basic setting and your desired colour of the crust—press start.

Nutrition:

Calories: 130 calories;

Total Carbohydrate: 25 g

Total Fat: 2 g

Protein: 3 g

CHAPTER 18:

Pleasure Bread

19.   Honey Beer Bread

Preparation Time: 2 hours

Cooking Time: 1 hour 20 minutes

Servings: 1½-pound loaf / 14 slices

Ingredients:

- 1 1/6 cups light beer, without foam

- Two tablespoons of liquid honey

- One tablespoon olive oil

- One teaspoon of sea salt

- One teaspoon cumin

- 2¾ cups bread flour

- 1½ teaspoons active dry yeast

Direction:

1. Prepare all of the ingredients for your bread and measuring means (a cup, a spoon, kitchen scales).

2. Carefully measure the ingredients into the pan.

3. Put all ingredients into a bread bucket in the right order, follow your manual for the bread machine.

4. Close the cover. Select the program of your bread machine to BASIC and choose the crust colour to MEDIUM.

5. Press START. Wait until the program completes.

6. When done, take the bucket out and let it cool for 5-10 minutes.

7. Shake the loaf from the pan and let cool for 30 minutes on a cooling rack.

8. Slice, serve and enjoy the taste of fragrant homemade bread.

Nutrition:

Calories 210; Total Fat 1.6g; Saturated Fat 0.2g; Cholesterol 0g; Sodium 135mg; Total Carbohydrate 42.3g; Dietary Fiber 1.8g; Total Sugars 2.6g; Protein 5.9g, Vitamin D 0mcg, Calcium 10mg, Iron 3mg, Potassium 91mg

CHAPTER 19:

Cakes and Quick Bread

20.   Cinnamon Pecan Coffee Cake

Preparation Time: 15 minutes

Cooking Time: 2 hours

Servings: 10 - 12

Ingredients:

- 1 cup butter, unsalted
- 1 cup of sugar
- Two eggs
- 1 cup sour cream
- One teaspoon vanilla extract
- 2 cups all-purpose flour
- One teaspoon baking powder
- One teaspoon baking soda
- 1/2 teaspoon salt
- For the topping:
- 1/2 cup brown sugar

- 1/4 cup sugar

- 1/2 teaspoon cinnamon

- 1/2 cup pecans, chopped

Directions:

1. Add butter, sugar, eggs, sour cream and vanilla to the bread maker baking pan, followed by the dry ingredients.

2. Select the Cake cycle and press Start, then Prepare toppings and set aside.

3. When the kneading cycle is done, about 20 minutes, sprinkle 1/2 cup of topping on top of the dough and continue baking.

4. During the last hour of baking time, sprinkle the remaining 1/2 cup of topping on the cake. Bake until complete. Cool it on a wire rack for 10 minutes and serve warm.

Nutrition:

Calories: 488 Cal

Sodium: 333 mg

Fiber: 2.5 g

Fat: 32.8 g

CHAPTER 20:

Meat Bread

21.   Collards & Bacon Grilled Pizza

Preparation Time: 15 minutes

Cooking Time: 15 minutes

Servings: 4

Ingredients:

- 1 lb. whole-wheat pizza dough

- 3 tbsps. garlic-flavoured olive oil

- 2 cups thinly sliced cooked collard greens

- 1 cup shredded Cheddar cheese

- ¼ cup crumbled cooked bacon

Directions:

1. Heat grill to medium-high.

2. Roll out dough to an oval that's 12 inches on a surface that's lightly floured. Move to a big baking sheet that's lightly floured. Put Cheddar, collards, oil, and dough on the grill.

3. Grease grill rack. Move to grill the crust. Cover the lid and cook for 1-2 minutes until it becomes light brown and puffed. Use

tongs to flip over the crust—spread oil on the crust and top with Cheddar and collards. Close lid and cook until cheese melts for another 2-3 minutes or the crust is light brown at the bottom.

4. Put pizza on the baking sheet and top using bacon.

Nutrition:

Calories: 498

Total Carbohydrate: 50 g

Cholesterol: 33 mg

Total Fat: 28 g Fiber: 6 g

Protein: 19 g Sodium: 573 mg

Sugar: 3 g Saturated Fat: 7 g

CHAPTER 21:

Multi-Grain Bread

22.   Baguette Style French Bread

Preparation Time: 2 hours

Cooking Time: 1 hour

Servings: 2 loaves

Ingredients:

- Two baguettes of 1-pound each
- Ingredients for bread machine
- One 2/3 cups water, lukewarm between 80 and 90 degrees F
- One teaspoon table salt
- Four 2/3 cups white bread flour
- Two 2/3 teaspoons bread machine yeast or rapid rise yeast
- Two baguettes of ¾-pound each
- Ingredients for bread machine
- One ¼ cups water, lukewarm between 80 and 90 degrees F
- ¾ teaspoon table salt
- 3 ½ cups white bread flour
- Two teaspoons bread machine yeast or rapid rise yeast

- Other Ingredients
- Cornmeal
- Olive oil
- One egg white
- One tablespoon water

Directions:

1. Choose the size of crusty bread you would like to make and measure your ingredients.
2. Add the ingredients for the bread machine to the pan in the order listed above.
3. Put the pan in the bread machine and close the lid. Switch on the bread maker. Select the dough setting.
4. When the dough cycle is completed, remove the pan and lay the dough on a floured working surface.
5. Knead the dough a few times and add flour if needed, so it is not too sticky to handle. Cut the dough in half and form a ball with each half.
6. Grease a baking sheet with olive oil. Dust lightly with cornmeal.
7. Preheat the oven to 375 **degrees** and place the oven rack in the middle position.
8. Using a rolling pin dusted with flour, roll one of the dough balls into a 12-inch by 9 -inch rectangle for the 2 pounds bread size or a 10-inch by 8-inch rectangle for the 1 ½ pound bread size. Starting on the longer side, roll the dough tightly. Pinch the ends and the seam with your fingers to seal. Roll the dough in a back

in forth movement to make it into an excellent French baguette shape.

9. Repeat the process with the second dough ball.

10. Place loaves of bread onto the baking sheet with the seams down and brush with some olive oil with enough space in between them to rise. Dust top of both loaves with a little bit of cornmeal. Cover with a clean towel and place in a warm area with any air draught. Let rise for 10 to 15 minutes, or until loaves doubled in size.

11. Mix the egg white and one tablespoon of water and lightly brush over both loaves of bread.

12. Place in the oven and bake for 20 minutes. Remove from oven and brush with remaining egg wash on top of both loaves of bread. Place back into the range, taking care of turning around the baking sheet. Bake for another 5 to 10 minutes or until the baguettes are golden brown. Let rest on a wired rack for 5-10 minutes before serving.

Nutrition:

Calories 87, Fat 0.8 g, carbs 16.5 g, sodium 192 mg, protein 3.4 g

CHAPTER 22:

Holiday Bread

23. Raisin Cinnamon Swirl Bread

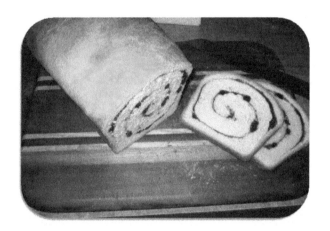

Preparation Time: 15 minutes

Cooking Time: 3 hours 35 minutes

Servings: 12

Ingredients:

Dough

- ¼ cup milk

- 1 large egg, beaten

- Water, as required

- ¼ cup butter, softened

- 1/3 cup white sugar

- 1 teaspoon salt

- 3½ cups bread flour

- 2 teaspoons active dry yeast

- ½ cup raisins

Cinnamon Swirl

- 1/3 cup white sugar

- 3 teaspoons ground cinnamon

- 2 egg whites, beaten

- 1/3 cup butter, melted and cooled

Directions:

1. For bread: Place milk and egg into a small bowl.

2. Add enough water to make 1 cup of mixture.

3. Place the egg mixture into the baking pan of the bread machine.

4. Place the remaining ingredients (except for raisins) on top in the order recommended by the manufacturer.

5. Place the baking pan in the bread machine and close the lid.

6. Select Dough cycle.

7. Press the start button.

8. Wait for the bread machine to beep before adding the raisins.

9. After Dough cycle completes, remove the dough from the bread pan and place onto lightly floured surface.

10. Roll the dough into a 10x12-inch rectangle.

11. For swirl: Mix together the sugar and cinnamon.

12. Brush the dough rectangle with 1 egg white, followed by the melted butter.

13. Now, sprinkle the dough with cinnamon sugar, leaving about a 1-inch border on each side.

14. From the short side, roll the dough and pinch the ends underneath.

15. Grease loaf pan and place the dough.

16. With a kitchen towel, cover the loaf pan and place in warm place for 1 hour or until doubled in size.

17. Preheat your oven to 350°F.

18. Brush the top of dough with remaining egg white.

19. Bake for approximately 35 minutes or until a wooden skewer inserted in the center comes out clean.

20. Remove the bread pan and place onto a wire rack to cool for about 15 minutes.

21. Cool bread before slicing

Nutrition:

Calories 297

Total Fat 10.6 g, Saturated Fat 6.3 g, Cholesterol 41 mg, Sodium 277 mg

Total Carbs 46.2 g, Fiber 1.7 g, Sugar 16.5 g, Protein 5.6 g

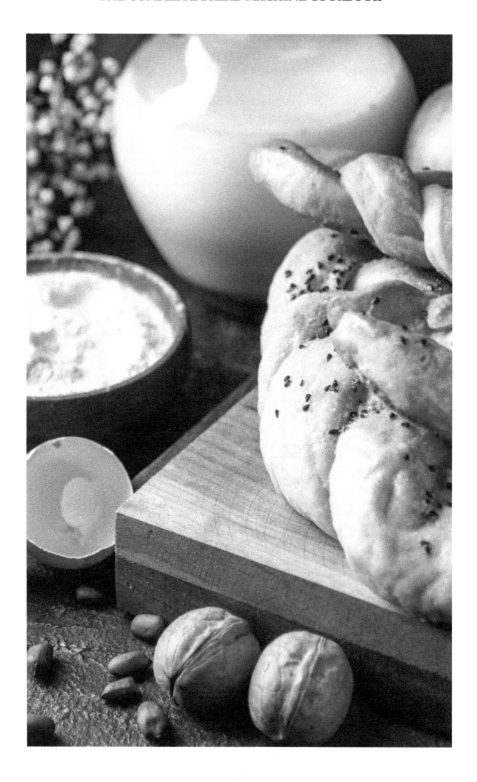

CHAPTER 23:

Keto Bread Recipes

24. Great flavor cheese bread with the added kick of pimento olives.

Preparation Time: 5 Minutes

Cooking Time: 3 Hours

Servings: 1 Loaf

Ingredients

- 1 cup water room temperature
- tsp. sugar
- 3/4 tsp. salt
- 1 ¼ cups shredded sharp cheddar cheese
- cups bread flour
- tsp. active dry yeast
- 3/4 cup pimiento olives, drained and sliced

Direction:

1 Add all ingredients except olives to machine pan.
2 Select basic bread setting.

3   At prompt before second knead, mix in olives.

Nutrition:

124 Calories,

4 g total fat (2 g sat. fat),

9 mg chol.,

299 mg sodium,

19 g carb. 1 fiber,

5 g protein

25. Ricotta Chive Bread

Preparation Time: 5 minutes

Cooking Time: 3 hours

Servings: 1 loaf

Ingredients:

- 1 cup lukewarm water
- 1/3 cup whole or part-skim ricotta cheese
- 1 ½ tsp. salt
- 1 tablespoon granulated sugar
- cups bread flour
- 1/2 cup chopped chives
- ½ tsp. instant yeast

Direction:

1 Add ingredients to bread machine pan except dried fruit.
2 Choose basic bread setting and light/medium crust.

Nutrition:

92 Calories,

0 g total fat (0 g sat. fat),

2 mg chol.,

207 mg sodium,

17 g carb. 1 fiber,

3 g protein

26. Red Hot Cinnamon Bread

Preparation Time: 5 minutes

Cooking Time: 3 hours

Servings: 1 loaf

Ingredients

- 1/4 cup lukewarm water
- 1/2 cup lukewarm milk
- 1/4 cup softened butter
- ¼ tsp. instant yeast
- 1 ¼ tsp. salt
- 1/4 cup sugar
- 1 tsp. vanilla
- 1 large egg, lightly beaten
- cups all-purpose flour
- 1/2 cup Cinnamon Red Hot candies

Direction:

1   Add ingredients to bread machine pan except candy.

2   Choose dough setting.

3   After cycle is over, turn dough out into bowl and cover, let rise for 45 minutes to one hour.

4   Gently punch down dough and shape into a rectangle.

5   Knead in the cinnamon candies in 1/3 at a t time.

6   Shape the dough into a loaf and place in a greased or parchment lined loaf pan.

7   Tent the pan loosely with lightly greased plastic wrap, and allow a second rise for 40-50 minutes.

8   Preheat oven 350 degrees.

9   Bake 30-40 minutes.

10 Remove and cool on wire rack before slicing.

Nutrition:

207 Calories,

6.9 g total fat (4.1 g sat. fat),

28 mg chol.,

317 mg sodium,

30 g carb. 1 fiber,

4.6 g protein

62. Cheddar Olive Loaf

CHAPTER 24:

International Bread

27.   Swedish Cardamom Bread

Preparation Time: 35 minutes

Cooking Time: 15 minutes

Servings: 1 loaf

Ingredients:

- ¼ cup of sugar

- ¾ cup of warm milk

- ¾ teaspoon cardamom

- ½ teaspoon salt

- ¼ cup of softened butter

- One egg

- Two ¼ teaspoons bread machine yeast

- 3 cups all-purpose flour

- Five tablespoons milk for brushing

- Two tablespoons sugar for sprinkling

Directions:

1. Put everything (except milk for brushing and sugar for sprinkling) in the pan of your bread machine.

2. Select the dough cycle. Hit the start button. You should have an elastic and smooth dough once the process is complete. It should be double in size.

3. Transfer to a lightly floured surface.

4. Now divide into three balls. Set aside for 10 minutes.

5. Roll all the balls into long ropes of around 14 inches.

6. Braid the shapes. Pinch ends under securely and keeps on a cookie sheet. You can also divide your dough into two balls. Smooth them and keep on your bread pan.

7. Brush milk over the braid. Sprinkle sugar lightly.

8. Now bake in your oven for 25 minutes at 375 degrees F (190 degrees C).

9. Take a foil and cover for the final 10 minutes. It's prevents over-browning.

10. Transfer to your cooling rack.

Nutrition:

Calories 135, Carbohydrates 22g, Total Fat 7g, Cholesterol 20mg, Protein 3g, Fiber 1g, Sugar 3g, Sodium 100mg

CHAPTER 25:

Fruit and Vegetable Bread

28. Blueberry Bread

Preparation Time: 3 hours 15 minutes

Cooking Time: 40- 45 minutes

Servings: 1 loaf

Ingredients:

- 1 1/8 to 1¼ cups Water
- 6 ounces Cream cheese, softened
- 2 tablespoons Butter or margarine
- ¼ cup Sugar
- 2 teaspoons Salt
- 4½ cups Bread flour
- 1½ teaspoons Grated lemon peel
- 2 teaspoons Cardamom
- 2 tablespoons Nonfat dry milk
- 2½ teaspoons Red star brand active dry yeast
- 2/3 cup dried blueberries

Directions:

1. Place all Ingredients except dried blueberries in bread pan, using the least amount of liquid listed in the recipe. Select light crust setting and the raisin / nut cycle. Press the start button.

2. Watch the dough as you knead. After 5 to 10 minutes, if it is dry and hard or if the machine seems to strain to knead it, add more liquid 1 tablespoon at a time until the dough forms a ball that is soft, tender, and slightly sticky to the touch.

3. When stimulated, add dried cranberries.

4. After the bake cycle is complete, remove the bread from the pan, place on the cake and allow to cool.

Nutrition:

Calories: 180 calories

Total Carbohydrate: 250 g

Fat: 3 g

Protein: 9 g

29. Pineapple Coconut Bread

Preparation Time: 10 Minutes

Cooking Time: 25 Minutes

Servings: 8

Ingredients:

- Six tablespoons butter, at room temperature
- Two eggs, at room temperature
- ½ cup coconut milk, at room temperature
- ½ cup pineapple juice, at room temperature
- 1 cup of sugar
- 1½ teaspoons coconut extract
- 2 cups all-purpose flour
- ¾ cup shredded sweetened coconut
- One teaspoon baking powder
- ½ teaspoon salt

Directions:

1. Preparing the Ingredients. Place the butter, eggs, coconut milk, pineapple juice, sugar, and coconut extract in your Hamilton Beach bread machine.

2. Select the Bake cycle. Program the machine for Rapid bread and press Start. While the wet ingredients are mingling, stir together

the flour, coconut, baking powder, and salt in a small bowl. After the first mixing is done and the machine motions, add the dry ingredients. When the loaf is done, eliminate the bucket from the machine. Let the loaf cool for 5 minutes. Slightly shake the pot to remove the loaf and turn it out onto a rack to cool.

Nutrition:

Calories 277

Cholesterol 9g

Carbohydrate 48.4g

Dietary Fiber 1.9g

Sugars 3.3g

Protein 9.4g

CHAPTER 26:

White Bread

30. Soft White Bread

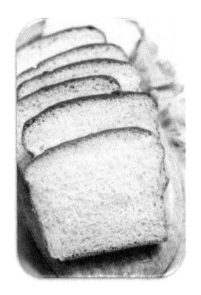

Preparation Time: 5 minutes

Cooking Time: 3 hours

Servings: 14

Ingredients:

- 2 cups water

- 4 teaspoon yeast

- 6 Tablespoon sugar

- ½ cup vegetable oil

- 2 teaspoon salt

- 3 cups strong white flour

Directions:

1. Add each ingredient to the bread machine in the order and at the temperature recommended by your bread machine manufacturer.

2. Close the lid, select the basic bread, low crust setting on your bread machine, and press start.

3. When the bread machine has finished baking, remove the bread and put it on a cooling rack.

Nutrition:

Carbs: 18 g

Fat: 1 g

Protein: 4 g

Calories: 74

CHAPTER 27:

Special Bread Recipes

31. Gluten-Free Peasant Bread

Preparation Time: 10 Minutes

Cooking Time: 25 Minutes

Servings: 8

Ingredients:

- 2 cups brown rice flour
- 1 cup potato starch
- 1 tbsp. xanthan gum
- 2 tbsp. sugar
- 2 tbsp. yeast (bread yeast should be gluten-free, but always check)
- 3 tbsp. vegetable oil
- Five eggs
- 1 tsp. white vinegar

Directions:

1. Preparing the Ingredients. Bloom the yeast in water with the sugar for five minutes.

2. Place all ingredients in the Cuisinart bread pan in the yeast-liquid-dry layering.

3. Put the pan in the Cuisinart bread machine.

4. Select the Bake cycle. Choose Gluten Free. Press start and stand by until the loaf is cooked.

5. The machine will start the keep warm mode after the bread is complete.

6. Let it stay in that mode for approximately 10 minutes before unplugging.

7. Remove the pan and let it cool down for about 10 minutes.

Nutrition:

Calories: 151

Sodium: 265 mg

Dietary Fiber: 4.3 g

Fat: 4.5 g

Carbs: 27.2 g

Protein: 3.5 g

32. Gluten-Free Hawaiian Loaf

Preparation Time: 10 Minutes

Cooking Time: 25 Minutes

Servings: 8

Ingredients:

- 4 cups gluten-free four
- 1 tsp. xanthan gum
- 2 1/2 tsp. (bread yeast should be gluten-free, but always check)
- 1/4 cup white sugar
- 1/2 cup softened butter
- One egg, beaten
- 1 cup fresh pineapple juice, warm
- 1/2 tsp. salt
- 1 tsp. vanilla extract

Directions:

1. Place all ingredients in the Cuisinart bread pan in the liquid-dry-yeast layering.
2. Put the pan in the Cuisinart bread machine.
3. Select the Bake cycle. Choose Gluten Free. Press open and wait until the loaf is cooked.

4. The machine will start the keep warm mode after the bread is complete.

5. Let it stay in that mode for 10 minutes before unplugging.

6. Remove the pan and let it cool down for about 10 minutes.

Nutrition:

Calories: 151

Sodium: 265 mg

Dietary Fiber: 4.3 g

Fat: 4.5 g

Carbs: 27.2 g

Protein: 3.5 g

CHAPTER 28:

Rolls and Pizza

33. Cheese Stuffed Garlic Rolls

Preparation Time: 5 Minutes

Cooking Time: 25 Minutes

Servings: 4

Ingredients:

- 3.2 cup bread flour
- 1.2 teaspoons salt
- 2 teaspoons granulated sugar
- 2.2 teaspoons olive oil
- 1 cup warm water
- 1 package active dry yeast
- 4 stick mozzarella string cheese sticks
- 0.5 stick melted butter
- 1 garlic salt

Directions:

1. Heat the water
2. Add yeast and stir

3. Let sit for 10 minutes

4. Pour yeast mixture in the bread pan

5. Add sugar, flour, oil and salt

6. Set machine to the dough cycle

7. Let the cycle finish

8. Remove from bread pan after the first rise

9. Knead dough until no longer sticky on a floured surface

10. Cut cheese sticks into 4 equal size pieces

11. Pinch off dough pieces and place a cut piece of cheese into center

12. Form ball around the cheese

13. After cheese is secured, edges sealed, roll the ball to form a rounder ball

14. Spray non-stick cooking spray on a pan

15. Place each ball about an inch apart

16. Cover, let rise until doubled

17. Preheat oven to 345°F after dough has risen

18. Bake for 15-20 minutes

19. Mix melted butter and garlic

20. Brush this mix over hot rolls

21. Serve with pizza or spaghetti sauce

Nutrition:

Carbs – 28 G, Fat – 3 G, Protein – 6 G, Calories – 160

CHAPTER 29:

Italian Styled

34. Veggie Loaf

Preparation Time: 20 minutes

Cooking Time: 0

Servings: 20

Ingredients:

- 1/3 cup coconut flour
- tablespoons chia Seed
- tbsps. psyllium husk powder
- ¼ cup sunflower seeds
- ¼ cup pumpkin seeds
- tbsp. flax seed
- 1 cup almond flour
- 1 cup zucchini, grated
- eggs
- ¼ cup coconut oil, melted
- 1 tbsp. paprika

- tsp cumin

- tsp baking powder

- tsp salt

Directions:

1. Grate carrots and zucchini, use a cheesecloth to drain excess water, set aside.

2. Mix eggs and coconut oil into bread machine pan.

3. Add the remaining ingredients to bread pan.

4. Set bread machine to quick bread setting.

5. When the bread is done, remove bread machine pan from the bread machine.

6. Cool to some extent before transferring to a cooling rack.

7. You can store your veggie loaf bread for up to 5 days in the refrigerator, or you can also be sliced and stored in the freezer for up to 3 months.

Nutrition:

Calories: 150

Carbohydrates: 3g

Protein: 3g

Fat: 14g

35.   Cajun Veggie Loaf

Preparation Time: 15 minutes

Cooking Time: 0

Servings: 12

Ingredients:

- ½ cup water
- ¼ cup onion, chopped
- ½ cup green bell pepper, chopped
- tsp garlic, chopped finely
- tsp ghee
- cups almond flour
- 1 tbsp. inulin
- 1 tsp Cajun seasoning
- 1 tsp active dry yeast

Directions:

1   Add water and ghee to bread machine pan.
2   Add in the remaining ingredients.
3   Set bread machine to basic setting.
4   When done, remove from bread machine and allow to cool before slicing.

5   Cool to some extent before transferring to a cooling rack.

6   You can store your bread for up to 5 days in the refrigerator.

Nutrition:

Calories: 101

Carbohydrates: 6g

Protein: 4g

Fat: 8g

36. Parmesan Italian Bread

Preparation Time: 16 minutes

Cooking Time: 0

Servings: 10

Ingredients:

- 1 1/3 cup warm water
- tbsps. olive oil
- cloves of garlic, crushed
- 1 tbsp. basil
- 1 tbsp. oregano
- 1 tbsp. parsley
- cups almond flour
- 1 tbsp. inulin
- ½ cup parmesan cheese, grated
- 1 tsp active dry yeast

Directions:

- Dispense all wet ingredients into bread machine pan.
- Add all dry ingredients to pan.
- Set bread machine to French bread.
- When the bread is done, remove bread machine pan from the bread machine.

- Cool to some extent before transferring to a cooling rack.

- You can store your bread for up to 7 days.

Nutrition:

Calories: 150

Carbohydrates: 14g

Protein: 5g

Fat: 5g

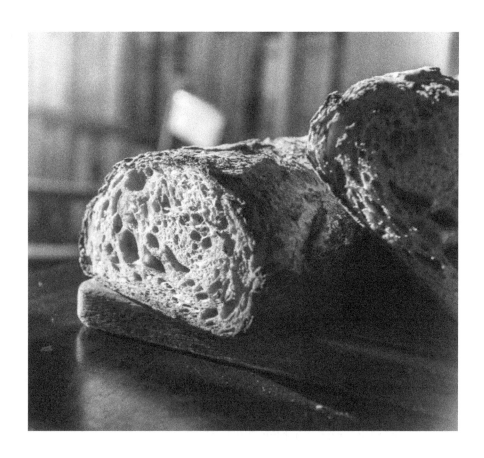

CHAPTER 30:

Famous Bread Recipes

37.   Best Keto Bread

Preparation Time: 10 minutes

Cooking Time: 30 minutes

Servings: 20

Ingredients:

- 1 ½ cup almond flour
- drops liquid stevia
- 1 pinch Pink Himalayan salt
- ¼ tsp. cream of tartar
- tsp. baking powder
- ¼ cup butter, melted
- large eggs, separated

Directions:

1   Preheat the oven to 375F.
2   To the egg whites, add cream of tartar and beat until soft peaks are formed.

3   Using a food processor, combine stevia, salt, baking powder, almond flour, melted butter, 1/3 of the beaten egg whites, and egg yolks. Mix well.

4   Then add the remaining 2/3 of the egg whites and gently process until fully mixed. Don't over mix.

5   Lubricate a (8 x 4) loaf pan and pour the mixture in it.

6   Bake for 30 minutes.

7   Enjoy.

Nutrition:

Calories: 90

Fat: 7g

Carb: 2g

Protein: 3g

38. Bread De Soul

Preparation Time: 10 minutes

Cooking Time: 45 minutes

Servings: 16

Ingredients:

- ¼ tsp. cream of tartar
- ½ tsp. baking powder
- 1 tsp. xanthan gum
- 1/3 tsp. baking soda
- ½ tsp. salt
  - 2/3 cup unflavored whey protein
- ¼ cup olive oil
- ¼ cup heavy whipping cream
  - drops of sweet leaf stevia
  - eggs
- ¼ cup butter
- oz. softened cream cheese

Directions:

1 Preheat the oven to 325F.
2 Using a bowl, microwave cream cheese and butter for 1 minute.
3 Remove and blend well with a hand mixer.
4 Add olive oil, eggs, heavy cream, and few drops of sweetener and blend well.

5   Blend the dry ingredients in another bowl.

6   Mix the wet ingredients with the dry ones and mix using a spoon. Don't use a hand blender to avoid whipping it too much.

7   Lubricate a bread pan and pour the mixture into the pan.

8   Bake in the oven until golden brown, about 45 minutes.

9   Cool and serve.

Nutrition:

Calories: 200

Fat: 15.2g

Carb: 1.8g

Protein: 10g

39. Chia Seed Bread

Preparation Time: 10 minute

Cooking Time: 40 minutes

Servings: 16 slices

Ingredients:

- ½ tsp. xanthan gum
- ½ cup butter
- 2Tbsp. coconut oil
- 1Tbsp. baking powder
- 3Tbsp. sesame seeds
- 2Tbsp. chia seeds
- ½ tsp. salt
- ¼ cup sunflower seeds
- cups almond flour
- 7eggs

Directions:

1 Preheat the oven to 350F.

2 Using a bowl, beat eggs on high for 1 to 2 minutes.

3 Beat in the xanthan gum and combine coconut oil and melted butter into eggs, beating continuously.

4 Set aside the sesame seeds, but add the rest of the ingredients.

5   Line a loaf pan with baking paper and place the mixture in it. Top the mixture with sesame seeds.

6   Bake for 35 to 40 minutes until a toothpick inserted comes out clean.

Nutrition:

Calories: 405

Fat: 37g

Carb: 4g

Protein: 14g

40. Special Keto Bread

Preparation Time: 15 minutes

Cooking Time: 40 minutes

Servings: 14

Ingredients:

- 2tsp. baking powder
- ½ cup water
- 1Tbsp. poppy seeds
- 2cups fine ground almond meal
- 5large eggs
- ½ cup olive oil
- ½ tsp. fine Himalayan salt

Directions:

1   Preheat the oven to 400F.
2   Using a bowl, combine salt, almond meal, and baking powder.
3   Drip in oil while mixing, until it forms a crumbly dough.
4   Make a little round hole in the middle of the dough and pour eggs into the middle of the dough.
5   Pour water and whisk eggs together with the mixer in the small circle until it is frothy.
6   Start making larger circles to combine the almond meal mixture with the dough until you have a smooth and thick batter.
7   Line your loaf pan with parchment paper.

8   Dispense batter into the prepared loaf pan and sprinkle poppy seeds on top.

9   Bake in the oven for 40 minutes in the center rack until firm and golden brown.

10   Cool in the oven for 30 minutes.

11   Slice and serve.

Nutrition:

Calories: 227

Fat: 21g

Carb: 4g

Protein: 7g

Conclusion

I n this book, we have discussed all bread machines and how we can put them to good use. Basic information about flour and yeast is also discussed to give all the beginners an idea of how to deal with the major ingredients of bread and what variety to use to get a particular type of bread. And finally, some delicious bread recipes were shared so that you can try them at home!

These loaves of bread are made using the everyday ingredients you can find locally, so there's no need to order anything or go to any specialty stores for any of them.

With these pieces of bread, you can enjoy the same meals you used to enjoy but stay on track with your diet as much as you want.

Moreover, we have learned that the bread machine is a vital tool to have in our kitchen. It is not that hard to put into use. All you need to learn is how it functions and what its features are. You also need to use it more often to learn the dos and don'ts of using the machine.

The bread machine comes with instructions that you must learn from the manual to use it the right way. There is a certain way of loading the ingredients that must be followed, and the instructions vary according to the make and the model.

So, when you first get a machine, sit down and learn the manual from start to finish; this allows you to put it to good use and get better results. The manual will tell you exactly what to put in it, as well as the correct settings to use, according to the different ingredients and the type of bread you want to make.

Having a bread machine in your kitchen makes life easy. Whether you are a professional baker or a home cook, this appliance will help you get the best bread texture and flavors with minimum effort.

Bread making is an art, and it takes extra care and special technique to deal with a specific type of flour and bread machine that enables you to do so even when you are not a professional.

Conversion Tables

Measuring Equivalent Chart

3 teaspoons	1 tablespoon
2 tablespoons	1 ounce
4 tablespoons	¼ cup
8 tablespoons	½ cup
16 tablespoons	1 cup
2 cups	1 pint
4 cups	1 quart
4 quarts	1 gallon

Type	Imperial	Imperial	Metric
Weight	1 dry ounce		28g
	1 pound	16 dry ounces	0.45 kg
Volume	1 teaspoon		5 ml
	1 dessert spoon	2 teaspoons	10 ml
	1 tablespoon	3 teaspoons	15 ml
	1 Australian tablespoon	4 teaspoons	20 ml
	1 fluid ounce	2 tablespoons	30 ml
	1 cup	16 tablespoons	240 ml
	1 cup	8 fluid ounces	240 ml
	1 pint	2 cups	470 ml
	1 quart	2 pints	0.95 l
	1 gallon	4 quarts	3.8 l
Length	1 inch		2.54 cm

* Numbers are rounded to the closest equivalent

Gluten-Free – Conversion Tables

All-Purpose Flour	Rice Flour	Potato Starch	Tapioca	Xanthan Gum
½ cup	1/3 cup	2 tablespoons	1 tablespoon	¼ teaspoon
1 cup	½ cup	3 tablespoons	1 tablespoon	½ teaspoon
¼ cup	¾ cup	1/3 cup	3 tablespoons	2/3 teaspoon
1 ½ cup	1 cup	5 tablespoons	3 tablespoons	2/3 teaspoon
1 ¾ cup	1 ¼ cup	5 tablespoons	3 tablespoons	1 teaspoon
2 cups	1 ½ cup	1/3 cup	1/3 cup	1 teaspoon
2 ½ cups	1 ½ cup	½ cup	¼ cup	1 1/8 teaspoon
2 2/3 cups	2 cups	½ cup	¼ cup	1 ¼ teaspoon
3 cups	2 cups	2/3 cup	1/3 cup	1 ½ cup

Flour: Quantity and Weight

Flour Amount
1 cup = 140 grams
3/4 cup = 105 grams
1/2 cup = 70 grams
1/4 cup = 35 grams

Sugar: Quantity and Weight

Sugar
1 cup = 200 grams
3/4 cup = 150 grams
2/3 cup = 135 grams
1/2 cup = 100 grams
1/3 cup = 70 grams
1/4 cup = 50 grams

Powdered Sugar
1 cup = 160 grams
3/4 cup = 120 grams
1/2 cup = 80 grams
1/4 cup = 40 grams

Cream: Quantity and Weight

Cream Amount
1 cup = 250 ml = 235 grams
3/4 cup = 188 ml = 175 grams
1/2 cup = 125 ml = 115 grams
1/4 cup = 63 ml = 60 grams
1 tablespoon = 15 ml = 15 grams

Butter: Quantity and Weight

Butter Amount
1 cup = 8 ounces = 2 sticks = 16 tablespoons =230 grams
1/2 cup = 4 ounces = 1 stick = 8 tablespoons = 115 grams
¼ cup = 2 ounces = ½ stick = 4 tablespoons= 58 grams

Oven Temperature Equivalent Chart

Fahrenheit (°F)	Celsius (°C)	Gas Mark
220	100	
225	110	1/4
250	120	1/2
275	140	1
300	150	2
325	160	3
350	180	4
375	190	5
400	200	6
425	220	7
450	230	8
475	250	9
500	260	

* Celsius (°C) = T (°F)-32] * 5/9

** Fahrenheit (°F) = T (°C) * 9/5 + 32

*** Numbers are rounded to the closest equivalent

CPSIA information can be obtained
at www.ICGtesting.com
Printed in the USA
BVHW010733270521
608096BV00018B/401